MW01503753

listening to silence

reflections of a pediatrician

Enjoy!
James McCrory 8/23/23

james hollis mccrory md

silent reflections
publishing and symposia
augusta, georgia

silent reflections
publishing and symposia
PO box 6654
augusta, georgia usa 30916

ISBN: 979883967715
library of congress control number: pending

front cover photo by S. Hermann and F. Richter
permission requested

back cover photo by Johannes Plenio
coolfreepix.com

cover design by Amber Lauwers

Prologue

it feels like horses running around in my chest
8-year-old with supraventricular tachycardia
a rapid, recurrent dysrhythmia

      Every dis---ease begins with a single symptom, generated by some troubled part of the anatomy. In 1938, George Burch at Tulane Medical School wrote an article in the journal Chest, correlating the chest pain known as angina pectoris to coronary artery disease. This observation forever linked the symptom to the underlying pathology. Some symptoms are precise. Others are vague. All point to disease.

      In the spring of 1974, a surgeon with a general practice in New Orleans offered an elective course in medical hypnotherapy. Sixteen out of a possible 592 medical students enrolled in the class. He offered insight in the semantics of symptoms and how they arise from the unconscious mind. His teachings included:

listen to the entire chief complaint
do not interrupt it
write it down, verbatim, in quotation marks

there is one word in the chief complaint
that points to the final diagnosis

once you make the final diagnosis
go back to the chief complaint
and underline that one word

if there is a sigh in the chief complaint
notate its exact location with an -s-

the closer the sigh is to the beginning
of the sentence
the greater the emotional burden
on the patient
the more likely the illness is psychosomatic

dedicated to

the wise clinician
and
the inquisitive patients

and to

the fine, gentle art
of being there
in silence

1

in the beginning
there is silence

silence is more than the mere absence of sound
it is the profound source
of all feeling and ideas

and words

silence is transparent

it is best appreciated
in quiet times
in the dark or twilight hours

in contemplative moments
without words

every story begins
with a single word

first words are important

especially the one word
which reveals the motive

whether a spiritual masterpiece
an epic poem
a novel
a play
a song
     or
a medical hi*story*

that word is an embryonic clue
pointing to the motive
which drives the story

it intrigues the listener

the wise listener
looks for that compelling word
in the opening lines of the narrative

every *dis---ease* begins with a single symptom
arising from some distempered part
disrupting silence

with time
the intensity crescendos to a point
that needs telling

the presenting symptom moves the afflicted
from solitude into relationship

someone becomes trusted
the symptom is told to another person

the quest for healing begins

4

before the compelling symptom is spoken
parallel lives exist

the clinician
contemplates the biological nature of diseases

somewhere else a patient suffers

healing begins
when the two are connected
by a call for help

silence is broken
a dialogue begins

whether spoken or implied

i need your help

are the four most important words
in any language

the three most powerful words are

i am here/hear

call and response

a plea goes out
an answer comes back
a connection is made

a dialogue begins

6

pathos   is suffering   in greek
logos   is word

path---ology is a word of suffering

clinicians in primary care
practice in clinics and emergency rooms

they see one patient at a time
every 10 to 30 minutes
4,000 to 7,000 times a year

they hear tens of thousands of symptoms annually
they dwell in a vast sea of complaints

most diagnoses in primary care
are based on symptomatology

the sooner that the first symptom is recognized
the earlier a diagnosis can be made

whether a common cold
a chronic ailment or
a rare disorder

medical caring begins
with a single symptom

7

the wise clinician
also listens to silence

looking for meaning
in pauses, hesitations, sighs
gasps and moans

8

inspiration occurs in silence
both figuratively and literally

from a newborn's first breath in
until our last breath out

our voices exist
only when we exhale

9

a newborn's first cry
is the first disruption of silence

it is a declaration
of want and need

     wwwaaaahhhhh

followed by a parental

     sssshhhhhhh

call and response

a primitive dialogue begins
without words

a relationship forms

the mother or father
soothes the infant

back into the comfort of silence

10

later
infants learn to   *coo*

vowels are born

    oooo 's

    aaahh's

    uuuuu's

    eeeee's

long liquid sounds
made without restricting the airways

mmm

about 6 months of age
consonants emerge
an infant begins to babble

coo-ing any vowel
with pursed lips
produces an
        mmm
the only bilabial consonant
made with both lips closed

not coincidentally
the word for mother in most languages
has an *m* in it

m's are soothing
they resonate from deep within
more than any other consonant
momma
home
oo*mmm*

mmm's come from so*m*e intangible location
there is no place like it

they are a vestigial link
to precognitive *m*emories

12

curious thing
   precognitive memories

contemplate them for a *mom*ent

approach them with preverbal sounds

   sssshhhh

   mmmm

13

infant babbling
with parental reinforcement
leads to mimicking

words are created
around 12 months of age
starting with

> *mama*
> *dada*

the primal relations

the next two words are

> *hi*
> *bye*

words of welcome and farewell
of coming and going
of recognition and affirmation

at 15 months of age
toddlers have 5-7 words

at 18 months
7-20 words

at 24 months
more than 50 words

words are combined
to make 2-3 word sentences

children entering kindergarten
with a larger vocabulary
do better in school

parents appreciate knowing this simple fact
especially those who have struggled in school as a kid

lap time reading with a child
does not last forever

yet it is spiritually more relevant
than all the child's future screen time

15

breathing occurs without thinking
99.999999% of the time

yet can be
brought into awareness
suddenly
with only a few words

words bring things
into consciousness

that is their job
that is what they do

that is their power

16

nonverbal sounds
persist throughout life
often quietly

sensitive parents and wise clinicians
perk up when they hear them and
explore their meaning

sighs originate and resonate from deep within
they point to
> unresolved emotions

> emerging grief

> unspoken misgivings

moans are nuanced

> *umm's*
>> show hesitation

>> half-formed concerns

> *huh's*
>> indicate emerging thoughts

>> newfound agreements

> *hmm's*
>> reveal a minor epiphany

>> an *aha!* lite moment

once upon a time...

children love stories
they are the source of
endless amazement and joy

opening words of a story are important
they set the mood
they frame the expectations
they introduce characters
they describe the motive
which drives the narrative

stories use words to document
what we know
what we believe

individually
they influence how a child learns

collectively
they create cultural identity

medically
*hi*stories are initially diagnostic and
ultimately therapeutic

educationally
a good teacher knows how an idea
can be is storied away into receptive minds
to last a lifetime
to be passed down through generations
to be recalled when needed

a parable becomes a paradigm

up…. up….up….

panted a frantic two-year-old

his shortness of breath and
distress was made worse
every time the doctor attempted to lay him flat
to listen to his heart

critical narrowing of the aortic valve
obstructs blood flow and
distends the ventricle and atrium

lung fluid accumulates
when left atrial pressure exceeds 26
well beyond the normal 2-5

adults in left sided heart failure
sleep upright on 1, 2 or 3 pillows
using gravity to shift lung fluid downwards
to relieve the feeling of suffocation

cardiologists call this orthopnea
from the greek

> *ortho---pnea*
> straight [up] breathing

> up…. up….up….

panted a two-year-old
telling the physician
he had   orth--***up***--nea

he did well postoperatively

water....water....water....

complained a two-year-old
in right sided congestive failure
from chronic lung disease due to prematurity

clinicians prescribe fluid restriction
for congestive heart failure

ever try explaining fluid restriction to a two-year-old
water....water....water....
biblically, fluid restriction is called thirsting

his 4 young siblings knew how to quiet him
by giving him water and quenching his thirst
mother got blamed for noncompliance and
rehospitalizations every couple of weeks
for recurrent heart failure

a decision was made to admit him
to the pediatric ward for 6 months
for fluid restriction
he was allowed to walk around the pediatric ward
on 25 yards of nasal oxygen tubing
a bit of free range
yet his exact location was always traceable

nurses, ward clerks, chaplains,
respiratory therapists, play therapists and
housekeepers took turns keeping him busy
during waking hours
it took a village to keep him distracted
from drinking water
4 months later   his heart failure resolved
he returned home to his mother and siblings

a good story is readily memorable and
quickly retrievable
unlike numerical data

a medical student
attends over 2400 hours of lectures and
pores over thousands of pathology slides, xrays,
images, charts, graphs and data

a well told patient history
can be brought back into memory by

    a simple word
    a phrase
    a feeling
    a memory
    a sensation
    a symptom

the story becomes real again
days, weeks, months, years or decades later

making a connection
so that an uncommon diagnosis
can be made

sometimes
in the blink of an eye

clinicians get to know their patients
by listening to their story and
how they tell it

in greek
gnosis   is knowledge
dia---gnosis is thorough knowledge
pro---gnosis is forward knowledge

first
patients volunteer a few symptoms

then
more symptoms are elicited
by asking specific questions

finally
the wise clinician probes the depths of silence
to form a more thorough knowledge
by repeating an open-ended question

      and what else.....

      and what else.....

      and what else.....

the full truth is hidden in silence
         and
requires trust, patience and opportunity
before revelation becomes possible

clinicians listen to symptoms and
look for physical signs

a murmuring heart
a wheezing lung

to make an initial impression
a clinical diagnosis
a working diagnosis

the final diagnosis may need confirmation by
        laboratory tests
        imaging studies
        biopsies
        physiologic studies

when you hear hoofbeats
on the pavement outside
 think first of horses
 not zebras

clinicians are taught this dictum early on

common conditions are easy to diagnose
rare ones are tricky

like hoofbeats
symptoms are only heard
never seen

there are hoofbeats and then there are hoofbeats

listening for the seldom heard but
distinct clippety-clop of a zebra hoof
is a learned skill

there are clues

the chief complaint is
the patient's first statement

wise clinicians treat the chief complaint
with utmost respect and
write it down verbatim

somewhere in the chief complaint
there is a word
that points to the final diagnosis

> *doctor, i have this chest pain whenever i......*

once the final diagnosis is made
the wise clinician goes back
to the chief complaint

and underlines the one word
that was there in the beginning
pointing to the final diagnosis

> *doctor, I have this chest <u>pain</u> whenever i......*

in greek
> *algia*   is pain

it is a compelling force
that drives a narrative

digressions are fun and instructive

> in the beginning
> there is a word
> that is different
> from all others
> it embodies the motive
> that drives the narrative
> the wise look for it

here are three famous first words in literature
two written by homer and one by moses
manin

> is the first word in greek literature
> the accusative form of
> *mania*
> usually translated as wrath

the wrath of achilles is the driving force
behind the epic poem *the iliad*
the trojan war lasted 10 years
because the enraged achilles
the strongest soldier
was humiliated in camp by agamemnon
before the troops set sail from aulis
acheilles refused to fight for a decade
until his friend patroclus was slain
he slew the trojan leader hector in revenge

the *motive* that drives the narrative
is tidily summed up in homer's first word
the first word in western literature

> *mania*

andra is the first word of homer's second epic *the odyssey*

      andra
      the man
      odysseus

hmm

      the protagonist
      the main character
      yet not a *motive*

odysseus was a sailor and a soldier
who fought 10 years in the trojan war and
wandered for another 10 years before returning home
to itacha

early on
there are clues to his *motive*
in line six
      noston   return
in line seven
      algia

he had a pain full of longing for a return home

in 1688 a swiss medical student johannes hofer
combined these two words into *nostalgia*
a painful homesickness
a morbid longing for a return to one's homeland
suffered by sailors, convicts and african slaves

an *algia* can be somatic or psychic in origin

an-algias are overprescribed
when psychological *algias* are ignored and
the patient's story is not fully told

glorifying men and war
homer produced two epic poems
containing 24 chapters each

amazingly
his 27,802 lines of dactylic hexameter
were passed down orally for 700 years
before being written down
by scribes in the library at alexandria

reflecting the silent capacity of
the human brain

one can only appreciate
the gift of idiot savants
in retaining huge volumes of verse and
passing it onto the next generation

more amazingly
regarding men and war
sitting bull once said

    a good warrior feeds his family

six words that redefine military purpose
to nurturing and survival of families
over property rights

beresith

is the first word in hebrew literature
which gets translated as
      genesis   in greek
      in principio   in latin
      in the beginning in english
hmm

      a very good place to start
      for an origin story
      yet   not a *motive*
   ruah   *moves*   across the face of the earth in line 6
   silently   inapparently
   atmospherically
   nourishing every living organism
   much like oxygen

the narrowest part
of the human airway
is the internal nares

when flow meets resistance
turbulence is created
a sound is produced
however subtle

in moments of quiet contemplation
a rush of air can be perceived
at the internal nares

like a symptom
ruah cannot be seen
it can only be heard
when one knows how to listen
during silent moments

a *sigh* is a rush of air
that fully expands the lungs
during an unanticipated deep breath

it opens tiny collapsed alveoli
improving oxygenation

it also indicates a deep emotion

when present in a chief complaint
a sigh is even more revealing than the key symptom

it signifies an anxiety or a hidden fear
whether stated or unstated
whether conscious or unconscious
whether known or unknown

it suggests the key symptom may be
       extraordinarily intense
       psychosomatic or
       like one in a relative with a fatal illness

the wise clinician explores the *sigh*
therein lies
the true purpose of the visit

even the location of the *sigh*
within the chief complaint
is significant

the wise clinician notates
its occurrence
with an   -s-

　　doctor, i have this chest <u>pain</u> -s- whenever I...

the closer the *sigh* is to the beginning of the sentence
the greater the patient's emotional burden
the more likely the nature of the illness is psychosomatic

towards the end of a patient's history
silent concerns need to be discovered
to reveal the untold parts of the story

and what else....

and what else....

and what else....

a repeated open-ended question

to be asked once trust has been established

three simple words that say

*i need to know more
so i can help you*

the complete story is revealed by probing silence

truth unfolds

33

a child brings a flower bud
to a pediatrician and asks

what kind of flower is this

i don't know

the child comes back the next day and
asks again

what kind of flower is this

oh, it's a rose

timing is important
in making a diagnosis

a child with unexplained fevers
may have normal laboratory tests for years
before juvenile rheumatoid arthritis
becomes diagnosable

a first-grade teacher requests an evaluation
for an intelligent 6-year-old
who is unmanageable and unteachable in the classroom

in the office
he climbs on the exam table
rips off the paper
jumps down
climbs up the sink
turns on the water
crawls into every conceivable space in the office
opens every drawer and cabinet
talks nonstop
otm otm: on the mind   out the mouth
no filters
no hidden agendas
just raw honesty and unbridled energy

when did you first notice he is hyperactive
pediatrician

in my 4th month
mother

in symptomatology
there are two critical points
on the timeline

when the patient perceives the earliest symptom and
when the key symptom is 1st reported to the clinician

the arc of the disease can be plotted by these 2 points

when a clinician encounters a patient
with already diagnosed chronic or rare illness
a key question is

what was the first thing you noticed was wrong

there is usually a moment of pause
for quiet reflection by the patient

many times
this question
has never been asked

patients are grateful for the opportunity
for a moment of reflection
to bring clarity and closure
regarding their initial quest for understanding

it also educates the clinician
to be a better listener
next time

weird symptoms are really annoying

they are disruptive to workflow on a busy day
a clinician can be readily at a loss
as to how to handle them

> *you can decide to hesitate*
> *but you can not hesitate to decide*
>   a wise surgeon

a lesser clinician ignores a weird symptom
which then frustrates and belittles the parent

a wise clinician is confused
but intrigued and
hears a zebra's clippety-clop

> *hmm*
> *this is unusual*
> *i need some time*
> *to think about this and*
> *get back to you*

the clinician openly decides to hesitate

the patient is relieved
having been heard and believed

the second point on the critical arc of
symptomatology has been satisfied

the symptom has been handed off
from patient to professional

the weirder the symptom
the rarer the zebra

>   *when i take him outside*
>   *he looks directly at the <u>sun</u>*
>   mother of a 6-month-old

this first symptom is highly unusual
it does not make immediate sense
it takes time to unravel

visual acuity is graded downwards from
            reading fine print to
            reading large print to
            finger counting to
            motion perception to
            light perception only

this infant was blind to the point of only
perceiving the brightest of all lights
the sun

he had sandifer's disease
a rare inborn error of metabolism
causing degeneration of the central nervous system

a new childhood cancer presents
approximately once
every 5000 pediatric visits

about once a year for clinicians
doing primary care of children only

perhaps one out of 50,000 to 100,000
symptoms heard annually

one study showed
a 12-14 week interval
between the initial presenting symptom and
the definitive diagnosis of a childhood cancer

with 4-5 visits
by one or more clinicians

clippety-clop   clippety-clop

   hmmm

what are the clues
to diagnose a childhood cancer
on the first examination

leukemias are the most common childhood cancers
white blood cells growing out of control
inside the bone marrow

when they reach a critical mass
they compress the periosteum
the inner lining of long bones
which contain pain fibers
the compression causes bone pain

the white cells growth also
crowds out the production of platelets
so easy bruising occurs

then as red cell growth is crowded out
the child becomes anemic
fatigue and paleness occur

any one of these symptoms alone
is not concerning

children play hard and
bump and bruise their legs all the time or
become anemic for lesser problems

a constellation of clinical findings
is concerning for leukemia

      bone pain
      easy bruising
      fatigue / paleness

all 3 cell lines in the bone marrow are involved

my leg is <u>stuttering</u>
                              a 5-year-old

his mother recalled his first words of concern

the family always went for a walk after dinner
junior fell behind
mom looked back and called out

what's wrong

junior described one-sided leg jerking
unilateral myoclonus
an upper motor neuron sign
pointing to a lesion in a muscle control area
of the central nervous system

he had a brain tumor

common symptoms are truly intense
when they are disabling to the point
of forcing the patient to bedrest

acute illnesses such as the flu last less than 2 weeks
subacute illnesses 2 to 12 weeks
chronic illnesses greater than 3 months

common symptoms extending
beyond the acute time frame
are concerning

my son has been vomiting
the doctors don't know what is wrong with him
the laboratory tests are normal
                    anxious mother, a physician

          don't worry about vomiting unless it has been
          at least 2 weeks
                    consulting pediatrician
                    in a distant city
it has been 3 weeks

          don't worry about prolonged vomiting
          unless he is having headaches

he is crying with severe headaches and can't sleep

          have your ophthalmologist friend examine his eyes
          if there is swelling of the optic nerves
          get a cat scan of his head

he had a brainstem tumor presenting with
vomiting, headaches and swelling of the optic nerve

2 common symptoms and a sign
a classical triad of obstruction of spinal fluid flow

brain tumors in the lower compartment of the skull
are the most common solid cancers of childhood

they present one of two ways
with muscle dysfunction or
obstructive hydrocephalus

the aim of education is simplification

this is especially true in medical education
so that a critical fact is readily remembered

in a crucial moment
crisis in greek was originally a legal term
referring to the final piece of evidence
that tipped the scales of justice
in one direction or another
towards guilt or innocence

around 400 bc
hippocrates adopted *crisis* as a medical term
to the critical moment in a disease
which influences the outcome of
either death or survival
due to limited therapies at the time
greek physicians were valued primarily
for two forms of knowledge
for diagnosis and prognosis

the *crisis* of an acute febrile illness
occurred on day 12
if the fever broke
it was called *lysis and*
the prognosis for survival was favorable
2420 years later
during the covid 19 pandemic
the *crisis* occurs on days 11-16

the chinese symbol for *crisis*
has a similar yet distinct dualistic meaning

危机

danger   opportunity

an elderly man could not remember
to take his blood pressure medicine twice a day

> *what is the last thing you do before you go to bed*

> *brush my teeth*

> *what is the first thing you do*
> *when you get up in the morning*

> *put on my shoes*

> *where should your medicine bottle be at night*

> *next to my toothbrush*

> *where should you put the bottle*
> *after you brush your teeth*

> *in my shoes*

> *what do you do with it after your morning dose*

> *put it by my toothbrush*

find a problem
fix a problem
with a brief, pragmatic action plan

in outpatient medicine
the *crisis* is distant
yet the importance of creating a turning point
is the same

a new mri scan costs $3,400,000
a new medical student costs $2,400,000 to educate

only one is sophisticated enough to
  listen
    inquire
      understand
        diagnose
          treat

a dying heart
needs one of two things
for resuscitation

usually it needs oxygen
to restore aerobic energy

occasionally it needs an electrical spark
to reset a functional rhythm

life support courses use the mnemonic   *ABC*
for airway, breathing, circulation
to prioritize the clinician's actions
in the *critical* moment

a more physiologically precise acronym is   *VOP*
for ventilation, oxygenation and perfusion

this triad is paired with 3 basic physical signs

ventilation	chest rise
oxygenation	pink
perfusion	palpable distal pulse

as both assessment of the situation and
therapeutic goals of restoration

better still than advanced resuscitation techniques
is anticipating and preventing
the cardiopulmonary arrest
by recognizing when the patient is
in respiratory failure or shock

my baby can't breathe
the intensity with which the parent says
the chief complaint
varies with the severity of illness

usually
this complaint means a newborn has a first cold and
nasal congestion is causing discomfort
from minor airway obstruction

the parent needs reassurance
the infant needs saline nose drops and suction

there is a continuum of respiratory symptoms
from distress to failure to arrest

with an increased work of breathing and facial distress

my baby can't breathe!

can mean impending respiratory failure
from critical airway obstruction
so that a call goes out to 911

the first symptom must be compelling
for the 911 system to be activated

> a mother walked 45 minutes in 1984
> to the emergency room with her infant
> she knew he was bad sick

on arrival
he was cold, blue and in shock
his condition was critical
the baby required massive
intravenous fluid resuscitation
he survived intact
an arrest was prevented

> *hmmm...... why didn't the mother call 911*
> thought the clinician

the infant was in shock
the mother's only symptom was not compelling

> *my baby is sleeping*

there are two outside doors
into every emergency room
one for ambulances
one for walk-ins
except for shock from trauma
this mother taught the clinician
that pediatric shock is a walk-in disease

hopefully the first person the parent sees
is the triage nurse versus a registration clerk
this mother did the right thing
the situation was critical
she got her infant there as fast as she could
she saved her baby's life

vague symptoms need immediate clarification

   my child is acting funny

a behavioral disturbance
needs differentiation
from a true medical emergency

   does your child recognize you

is a precise question
looking for an altered mental status
which can lead to coma due to
        respiratory failure
        shock
        seizures
        central nervous system disease

there is only one right answer to the question
        does your child recognize you
an immediate   *yes*
without doubtful modifiers
        sort of   kind of
        maybe   I think so
        i guess   y y...yes...
common qualifiers sound like weak positives
wise clinicians treat them like strong negatives
even
        [a pause to thing about the answer....]
is a strong negative

a child who fails to recognize the parents
is in eminent medical danger
failure to recognize parents is the symptom
lack of eye contact with parents is the sign

50

words are like numbers
                    george burch md

words mean what you want them to mean
                    lewis g carrol

truth lies somewhere between
the precision and the vagueness of symptoms

        doctor, I have chest pain
                [indicates with clenched fist over sternum]

        doctor, I don't feel well

in 1938
george burch wrote an article
in the journal chest
correlating angina pectoris
with coronary artery disease

brilliantly linking the symptom
to the underlying pathology and
changing the direction of cardiology

chest pain in an 11-year-old and a worried mother

> *my chest hurts*
>> a 6th grade boy

>> **where** *were you when it first hurt*
>>> clinician
> (puzzled look)
>> *at home or in school*

> *in school*
>> **where** *in school*
> *in the gym*
>> *what were you doing*
> *playing dodge ball*
>> *what were you doing when it first hurt*
> *sliding on the floor*

>> *oh*
>>> said the mother

differentiating somatic from psychosomatic pain
is important
people tend to forget when a chronic pain first occurred
asking   *did you hurt yourself*
leads to denial of forgotten minor trauma

memory is good at remembering
where you were at the time

recreating the scene gets to the diagnosis quickest
and helps separate somatic from psychosomatic pain

imaging studies for this symptom
would be nonrevealing

children spend most of their lives in a hypnotic state
they are very open to suggestions

surgeon with a general practice
in a neighborhood in new orleans
adjacent to the french quarter

he used medical hypnotherapy for
anesthesia for minor procedures
weight loss
smoking cessation
psychotherapy
he also offered this elective to medical students
once a year on his wednesday afternoons off
his teaching included

do not interrupt the chief complaint
write it down, verbatim, in quotation marks

sociologists have studied clinicians taking chief complaints
physicians interrupt it between the 6th and 7th second
physician assistants & nurse practitioners listen to all of it

there is one word in the chief complaint
that points to the final diagnosis

once you make a final diagnosis
go back to the chief complaint and underline that one word

if there is a sigh in the chief complaint
notate its exact location with an -s-

the closer the sigh is to the beginning of the sentence
the greater the emotional burden on the patient
the more likely the illness is psychosomatic

a clinician has about 20 minutes
to determine if a symptom is
psychic or somatic in origin

it is an important bifurcation

an untold story of stress
can lead to unnecessary tests

a presumptive diagnosis of anxiety
can lead to a delay in diagnosis
of an organic disease

what is the impact of [a common racial slur]
television interviewer

there is only one true pejorative
in the english language
the "s" word

it so disabling, so debilitating, so cruel
to call anyone stupid
especially a young girl
it leaves her defenseless

whoopi goldberg

at some point
tell every child:
you are smart
and can say
STOP!

there are only two kinds of questions
    asked questions
    unasked questions

the latter are dangerous
leading to false assumptions and misdirection

the aim of education is the same as
medical history taking
it is to create
a safe environment
for asked questions

there are no *''s----d''* word questions
there are only unsafe environments

young lady
don't you EVER!
say NO to me
or anyone else

words spoken in a rage to a child
can have a permanent effect

intimidation and violence
amplify the effect

children tend to believe
what they are told
especially when in a fugue state

hypnotic suggestions are powerful

emotional trauma can last longer
than physical trauma

it can leave a child defenseless and
a set up for a lifelong victimhood

when someone dies
the family members will keep the memory alive
by recreating the death scene
general surgeon
teaching medical hypnotherapy
hmmm
well that seems dubious
thought the medical student

15 years later, he is an attending physician and receives a late-night call from his senior resident

i have just admitted a 15-year-old girl
to the pediatric intensive care unit
she is having premature ventricular contractions
her uncle died two nights ago from a heart attack
in the intensive care unit just down the hallway
she drank a lot of coca colas at his wake
her caffeine level is high
causing her a few pvc's
oh by the way
she has been admitted to 3 other hospitals in the past
one for a laryngoscopy for hoarseness
one for a stomach endoscopy for upper abdominal pain
one for a colon endoscopy for lower abdominal pain
all tests were normal
senior resident
hmmm
thought the attending

death scene recreated
4th hospitalization in a healthy child
the symptom complex makes no anatomical sense
heart, vocal cords, stomach, colon

he instructs the senior resident
> *good diagnosis and treatment*
> *you have done everything right*
> *there is nothing more that needs done now*
> *oh by the way*
> *there is something psychosomatic going on here*
> *tell the mother that we spoke*
> *that her daughter is safe*
> *that I will see her first thing in the morning*
> *don't mention my psychosomatic concerns*

the senior resident tells this to the junior resident
who tells it to the medical student
who tells the mother
> *the attending isn't coming in tonight*
> *he says this is all psychosomatic*
> *he will see you in the morning*

the mother is livid the next morning
trying to control her rage
speaking through clinched teeth

> *-s- "doctor, I know you think this is psychosomatic*
> *but it isn't psychosomatic*
> *I have taken her to four different hospitals now*
> *and none of the doctors can tell me*
> *what is wrong with my daughter*
> *they did a laryngoscopy at hospital......"*

the chief complaint lasted 43 minutes
the pediatric attending did not interrupt
instead he reflected upon the general surgeon's teachings

the closer the sigh is to the beginning of the sentence
the greater the emotional burden
the more likely it is a psychosomatic illness
this sigh had even preceded the quotation marks
first time he had ever heard that
the symptom complex made no anatomical sense

the mother's pressured speech slowed down
37 minutes later
she realized that she was not going to be interrupted
for the first time ever
at 43 minutes she said

-s- doctor what do you think is wrong with my daughter

he responded hesitantly
mustering up courage to suggest a noxious diagnosis

-s- this may make you very angry
but a thought that occurred to me
while listening to you just now
i once admitted a 15-year-old girl
to this same room
several times in status epilepticus
i overmedicated her with multiple anticonvulsants
until I figured out she was having
pseudo-seizures to get away from her stepfather

tears began pouring from the mother's eyes
her stepfather had sexually abused her as a child and
was still in the household
abusing her daughter

the sigh before a 43-minute chief complaint and
a similar story
were the only clues

wart removal by application of liquid nitrogen
is a moderately painful procedure
even though there is no incision or injection
anticipation of the procedure is also
anxiety provoking in a child

dabbing on the liquid nitrogen
with a cotton swab initially lessons the pain and
numbs the area before a larger dose is used
by a jet spray on technique
is this going to hurt
   let me show you what i am going to do
    [using a dry swab for demonstration]
   i am going to count to ten
   dabbing this swab on once each time
   if this bothers you
   you say STOP
   and i will stop
   the first time
   right when you say stop
   do you understand

  yes
   good
   what do you say if it bothers you

  stop
   good
   and when do i stop
  right away
   good
   now lets practice this 1, 2, 3...

  stop
   good
   now a little louder this time 1, 2, 3, 4, 5...
  STOP!
   very good

is this going to hurt

is the unspoken fear in every child's mind
when talking to a clinician

hurt is a four lettered word

if no procedure is planned
the child needs reassurance
at the beginning of the visit

if there is an injection or procedure
the wrong answer is

> *no*
> *it's not going to hurt*

a child knows when pain
is compounded by a lie and
recognizes betrayal
future trust becomes shattered

the right answer is honest and
does not mention the *h* word

> *i am going to as gentle*
> *as I know how to be*
> *you let me know*
> *if this* **bothers** *you*

children are not allowed to cry
in the pediatric emergency room
sign in the staff lounge in 1980
at east tennessee childrens hospital

the intent of the sign
was to change the approach of clinical personnel
to the child

to center everything around the child's needs
from the child's perspective

children cry when threatened
abandoned or in pain

making a children's emergency room
welcoming and safe
takes foresight and planning

children need a safe refuge
filled with friends
they can trust

hannibal and his elephants
crossed the alps in 218 bc
his troops could not penetrate the walls of rome
even after a prolonged siege

instead
they marched southward and
decimated the advanced culture
of southern italy
which never recovered
rome grew in prominence thereafter

in the 1960s
an american latin professor
dining outdoors at a café
in a small village in southern Italy
watched a 2 year being
boisterous and disruptive
at his family's table

the italian grandmother got up
walked around to his chair and
whispered two words
into his ear

the boy became pale and silent and
quiet for the rest of the dinner
the parents did not hear the two words
the latin teacher did

hannibal's coming

over 2,000 years later through oral tradition
an emotional impact was made
historical trauma is real

    did you just have a nightmare
        mother of a teenager
        entering his room to wake him for school
          finding him pale and frightened
      yes

    i tell you what to do next time
    it is an easy trick
    just as soon as you figure out you are dreaming
    wake up and the nightmare will be gone

it worked

20 years later he is married and
wakes up with a nightmare
his wife walks in and asked

    did you just have a nightmare
        yes

    let me tell you a story
    once when i was a teenager
    i woke up frightened by a nightmare
    just as my mother walked in the room
    to get me up for school
    she spoke
        did you just have a nightmare
    yes

        let me tell you what to do next time
        as soon as you wake up
        go right back to sleep again
        and beat the hell out of 'em

a clinician meets a 13-year-old boy with autism
for the first time

the child is silent, detached and distant
looking down
with no eye contact
dressed kinda different

the clinician is unsure if he is verbal or intelligent
so he issues a challenge

> *can you say*
> *the quick brown fox jumped over the lazy dog*
> > *the quick brown fox jumped over the lazy dog*
>
> *good*
> *do you know what is unique about that sentence*
> > *no*
>
> *it has every letter in the alphabet in it*

the clinician uses that sentence as a test
of enunciation of 26 letters

detached silence again
no eye contact
two minutes later

> *there is no "s" in that sentence*

the clinician had said *jumped* instead of *jumps*
the correct sentence is
> *the quick brown fox jump**s** over the lazy dog*

touché
the clinician learned
underestimation is a form of prejudice

preventing teenage deaths

> *i am not a psychiatrist*
> *i am not a psychologist*
> *i am a preacher*
> *i don't know much about teenagers*
> *all I know is that they are still your children*
> *and you must keep them alive*
> > a preacher in the early 1950s

teenage black males are 6 times more likely
to be shot by a police officer
than teenage white males
> *don't wear a hoodie*
> *don't try to break up a fight*
> *don't talk back to cops*
> *don't ask for help*
> *don't give them an excuse to kill you*
> *i don't care about you're being right*
> *i just want to you to come home alive*
> > the talk given by parents
> > to teenage black sons

there is one death every 26 minutes
in the united states from drunk driving

> *to end drunk driving*
> *to help fight drugged driving*
> *to support the victims of these crimes and*
> *to prevent underage drinking*
> > mission statement
> > mothers against drunk driving

native americans aged 11 to 24
are 5 times more likely to commit suicide
than nonnative youths

what can one person do

montana has the highest suicide rate per capita
in the united states

a family practitioner in billings
specializes in addiction medicine
in the community clinic
in the inner city

her patients include homeless crystal meth addicts
who sleep in the snow in wintertime

she gives them her cell phone number
with the instruction

> *call me if you are ever thinking seriously*
> *about hurting yourself*

she gets a 2:30 am call about every 3 months and
directs the patient to a specified emergency room

the triage nurse greets them by name and
puts them at the head of the line

the family practice resident comes down and
admits the patient to the hospital

nice access to care

the easiest way to stop smoking is to never start

> *the single most important decision*
> *you make between ages 11 and 20*
> *is whether you use tobacco*
>> advice to preteens and teens
>> in front of parents
>
> *i am not going to tell you the right answer*
> *you are smart*
> *you already know the right answer*
> *i am only going to say*
> *that it is a decision only you can make*
>
> *i cannot make it for you*
>
> *your dad / mom really do not want you to smoke*
>> *and....*
>
> *they cannot make the decision for you*
> *part of growing up is making your own decisions*
> *about your own body*
>> *and....*
>
> *your friends can not make the decision for you either*
> *what is it called if your friends ask you to do*
> *something unhealthy*
>> *peer pressure*
>
> *and how do you handle peer pressure*
>> *i say no*
>
> *and you can be nonjudgmental when you say no*
> *they can smoke and be cool*
> *you can not smoke and be cool*
> *if you don't judge them, they can't judge you*
>> *and....*
>
> *i guarantee you in two years*
> *that they will be very unhappy with their decision*
>> *and*
>
> *you will be incredibly happy with yours*

i just really like my children's pediatrician
a retired third grade teacher
now a grandmother

why
asked the resident in training

he always writes his instructions
on a small piece of paper and
gives them to me
at the end of each visit
so when i get home
i remember everything he has told me to do

simple instructions
handwritten
are more powerful than a computer print out

it takes a good deal of thought
to simplify the complex

40 years later
the one-time resident
adds his cell phone number
to the bottom of the note
saying
text me if you have any questions about this or
if your child gets worse
a few times a week
he gets a text message back
asking for clarification
it usually takes 30 seconds or less

simple access
positive feedback

text messaging is more efficient than emails

the more employees an institution has
the less likely you are going to be
to get a human to answer a telephone call
much less find a person who can answer your question

frustrating   isn't it

businesses implement
time management techniques
to isolate employees
from interruptions
to improve productivity

these efforts backfire

harvard business review published
a counterintuitive article on managing interruptions
stating
> *the interruptions are your job*
> *deal with them*

this insight is reminiscent
of street wisdom
written on a teenager's t shirt

> *gravity sucks*
> *deal with it*
>> extreme punk skateboarder

time is valuable
so is access
texting saves time
for both patient and clinician

doctor -s- i don't know what is wrong with me

a sigh -s- points to anxiety

superficially
anxiety seems like fear lite
but fear is transient and protective

anxiety is far more permanent
pernicious and destructive

its chronicity leads to social withdrawal
obesity, hypertension, diabetes and
innumerable other diseases

valium was the number 1 selling pharmaceutical
in the united state
in the 1970s

there are healthier ways
of dealing with anxiety

awareness of breathing
encouragement of moving
are relaxing substitutes for stress

>   *breath deeper*
>   *move more*
>   *eat less*

tell me something
what is the appeal of crystal meth
                    pediatrician

first it takes away all of your anxieties
then it takes away everything else
                    16-year-old native american girl
                    in a juvenile detention center

she had been a straight a student
with a part time job and
a savings account

the clinician's reality
is not the patient's reality

the clinician's responsibility
is to create an atmosphere
conducive for the patient
to state their reality

without judgement

somatic diseases cause anxiety
anxiety causes psychosomatic symptoms

a clinician has about 20 minutes to distinguish
between the two

some patients are convinced
their symptoms are somatic in origin and
want elaborate testing

due diligence is always in order

other patients realize
stress and anxiety are the root cause
yet want the clinician to mention the possibility first
before they open up completely

between the 6th and the 12th minute of the exam
when anxiety is a likely etiology
the possibility needs to be broached

> *do you think stress can be an element here*
> *yes, i have been worried about......*

otherwise
the true purpose of the visit may only emerge
when the patient's hand reaches the door handle
and they say

> *oh, by the way*

a well-timed visit begins with a chief complaint and
ends with a pragmatic plan

comfort food is a euphemistic misnomer
stress eating is a more precise term

it leads to obesity
hypertension and diabetes mellitus

a successful baker in downtown atlanta
was famous for his sweet potato cheesecakes

even a president stopped by one day
to take one back to the first lady
in the white house

the baker's world consisted
mainly of butter
flour and sugar

when he reached 260 pounds
he developed diabetes

he lost 70 pounds
by altering his diet and exercise

he never took any medications

a 65-year-old reached 236 pounds and
became the first in the family
to develop diabetes

a clinician recommended
removing all white substances from the diet
     sugar   flour   milk
     bread   potatoes ice cream
     rice   grits
everything white
except for cauliflower
the patient lost 30 pounds

diet is the easiest and hardest thing to change
eliminating sugar and flour
can eliminate adult diabetes

criminal lawyers say that
the verdict is determined at jury selection
likewise   body size is determined
when food items are removed from a grocery shelf

it takes 21 days or to change a habit permanently
getting a patient to state their age in years
then committing to spend that many days
walking each day is a start
with the suggestion
       the more i move
       the better i feel
       the better i feel
       the more i move
with smaller incremental changes in diet
such as giving up snacking for 6 hours
then 12 hours
then 24 hours...

to build instant rapport with someone
look at their shoulders
look at their chest rise and
breath in sync with them
this will establish an unconscious connection
                    a hypnotherapist
         hmmm   sounds fishy
                    thinks the clinician
a few years later
the clinician awakens at 3 am and
cannot get back to sleep
he doesn't want to disturb his spouse
so he starts breathing in sync with his spouse
who also starts to breath deeper and slower
it was relaxing
then a few minutes later
he hears a third breath
from the small dog sleeping at their feet
3 deep breaths in sync while 2 of them were sound asleep
only time in 7 years that that he ever heard
his dog breath at night

he tells this story to the lieutenant colonel
in the workstation next to him
who tells him this story
              my 15-year-old dog is too big
              to get in bed
              so he sleeps beside me on the floor
              he has congestive heart failure and
              has a hard time breathing
              when i am tired and frazzled
              i lay down at night and
              breath in sync with him
              i am sound asleep in 5 minutes
              without a care in the world

an overworked x-ray technician
acts unprofessionally in a small inner city
pediatric intensive care unit

> *I just don't like her attitude*
> *she was just so rude and mean to us*
> *she has that old [public hospital] attitude*
>   senior ward clerk
> *you should call her and tell her*
>   pediatrician

she called and said
> *i don't like your personality*
> *the way you treated our patient and nurse...*

> *you need to call her back and apologize*
> *why*
> *i recommended a change in her attitude*
> *you attacked her personality*
> *that's unfair*
> *you and i have the same personality*
> *we have had since age two*
> *personality is not changeable*
> *attitude is*

the ward clerk immediately called back
the apology was accepted
after that, future x-rays were done quickly
with a smile from the young x-ray technician

in terms of fixing things in a 20-minute visit
the clinician can demonstrate how to change
                    attitude   behavior
                    posture   breathing pattern
this feels good
modeling immediate changes creates a pathway
to make permanent changes

for emotional wounds to heal
the patient needs
someone they trust to believe them

stories are how we struggle with adversity
resilience is how we overcome adversity
compassion is how we nurture resilience
forgiveness is how we move on

instead of criminal trials
nelson mandela and desmond tutu in south africa
established public forums for storytelling
of brutalities suffered during apartheid

prison guards listened to survivors
so that healing of both could begin

sudden traumatic events
can block proper memory formation

distorted memories prolong
post-traumatic stress
as can
>fear and shame
>overly protective loved ones
>misinformation
>unasked questions
>fear of retribution

a patient's story telling
in a safe
nonjudgmental
setting
can demystify false memories and
facilitate self-healing

how old are you?
                    pediatrician

            i have been here 72 winters
                    northern cheyenne grandmother 2014

she remembered her grandmother
who had been a child
camped with her mother
on the banks of the little bighorn river
on the morning of june 25, 1876
unaware of custer's approach

life on the northern plains has never been easy
 in 2015
the grandmother's 16-year-old granddaughter
became pregnant
the expectant mother had multiple health problems
the pediatrician was worried

        how is she going to handle this

                she is going to learn how to suffer

        oh

a few months later
the great-great-great-great granddaughter is born

mother and child are both healthy

on his last afternoon in a clinic
after 3.5 years on a native american reservation
a pediatrician picks up a chart
before going into the exam room

chief complaint: acne

he walks in and there is a teen-age girl
well dressed
with totally clear skin
sitting with her mother

> *uummm*
> *the chart here says acne*
> > *yes*
> > *i know*
> > *do you remember me*
> *refresh my memory*
> > *you used to come visit me every week*
> > *two years ago*
> > *when i was*
> > *in the juvenile detention center*
> *ahh yes*

he remembered her dressed in orange
during his weekly clinic there

once he had prescribed
face washes and cream for her acne

> *i heard you are leaving the reservation soon*
> *i just wanted to let you know before you go*
> *that i am graduating from high school*
> *in 2 months*

eskimos have 72 words for snow
they live in it

there are an infinite variety of silences
all sounds, words and stories originate from it

words bring things into consciousness
that is their power

this small tome has called attention
to symptoms and sighs arising from silence

to get to a *dia---gnosis*
a thorough knowledge

certain words are diagnostic
other words initiate healing

unlike eskimos
we are not surrounded by silence
we are silence deprived

we must actively seek
its passive beauty
by turning off electronic devices and
by putting down the book
dear reader

> *all beings arise from silence*
> *all beings return to it....*

About the author

James McCrory's passions are pediatrics, piano and philology. He has been involved in medical education for 50 years. He enjoys bringing innovative ideas to teaching the healing arts: especially using Socratic dialogue in small group discussions.

Beginning in the 8th grade at John Gorrie Junior High School in Jacksonville, Florida, and then at the Bolles School, he studied Latin for 9 years. He graduated from Vanderbilt University in 1972 with a major in Latin and a minor in Greek. He attended the American School for Classical Studies in Athens that summer.

James graduated from Tulane Medical School in 1976. After completing pediatric residency and fellowship training in Jacksonville, he practiced and taught pediatric critical care medicine for 32 years. He has served on faculties at the University of Florida, Mercer School of Medicine, Emory Medical School, Morehouse School of Medicine and Vanderbilt University.

He is a contributing editor to the original Pediatric Advanced Life Support [PALS] Course, published by the American Heart Association and the American Academy of Pediatrics in 1987. He trained national PALS faculties in the United States, India, the Philippines, Mexico, Malaysia, Belgium, England and Paraguay. Recently, James has practiced general pediatrics for the Indian Health Service on the Northern Cheyenne in Lame Deer, Montana, and for the Family Medicine Residency program at Eisenhower Medical Center on Fort Gordon, Georgia.

PLEASE HELP SPREAD THE WORD

via social media to your friends
via Facebook "likes"
at Dr James McCrory or Silent Reflections
sending gift copies to your favorite doctors,
nurses and physician assistant

doing literary readings at social gatherings
inquiring about translating into your native language
inquiring about sponsoring a translator into your
native language

james@silentreflections.org
                i need your help
                        jhm

Favorite quote: *a good warrior feeds his family*
                                Sitting Bull